The Mirror has Two Faces

Cally Bassage

Copyright © 2019 Cally Bassage

All rights reserved.

ISBN: 9781704735627

CONTENTS

Dedication

Prologue

Chapter 1 – Meeting Bipolar

Chapter 2 – The Rollercoaster Begins

Chapter 3 – Seeking Solutions

Chapter 4 – To and Fro

Chapter 5 – Hidden Gifts and Deep Despair

Chapter 6 – Highs and Hallucinations

Chapter 7 – Missing pieces

Chapter 8 – Looking Back

Chapter 9 – Hope

Chapter 10 – Family Support

Chapter 11 – Medical Memoirs

Chapter 12 – Living in the now

Chapter 13 – New Beginnings

GLOSSARY

POETRY

DEDICATION

I would like to dedicate this book to my family – Mom (Sue), Dad (Jack), my sisters Lilla and Bridget and my brother Derrin. They have seen me at my best and at my worst and always they believed that I would recover. Throughout all my ups and downs they have been there for me – supportive and encouraging. No-one can ask for more than that!

I offer my sincere thanks to the many doctors and nurses, psychiatrists and psychologists who specialise in understanding the deep mysteries of mental illness. It is a challenging job and for those of you who walk the road with us – you are a beacon of hope in a dark existence.

To Greg (my partner) for holding my hand and believing in me and offering me his unconditional love.

I would also like to thank the many people that have made this book possible. My co-writer Jenne Rennie who helped me make sense of my words and ideas and helped me put something tangible together. Thanks to my editor, Trish Beaver, who also nursed the book through its final stages.

I am grateful to my friends and family who have read the drafts and made constructive comments and suggestions. I really appreciate the effort.

Finally and most importantly my thanks and gratitude to God for without my faith in him I would surely have succumbed to the darkness.

PROLOGUE

"You have stories worth telling, memories worth remembering, dreams worth working toward, a body worth feeding, a soul worth tending and beyond that, the God of the universe dwells within you, the true culmination of super and natural."

- Danielle La Porte-The Fire Starter Session

I was the child who had it all. A comfortable home, loving parents, siblings, friends and extended family. I excelled at school, I excelled on the sports field, I was a cheerful outgoing attractive leader, I loved an audience and the world was there waiting for me. So what went wrong? Why did my life change? Why was confidence replaced with terror? How did this happen? How *could* this happen? Why did this happen? The answer to the last question is simple, I don't know and I won't ever know, but I do know it happens to other people more often than one would think. It is a journey no one would willingly take. Countless thousands of people are thrust into the unfamiliar territory of psychotic depression, their lives (and those of their families) upended and turned into chaos. A future that once seemed secure and bright suddenly becomes dark and fraught with terror.

This is a book about my journey – my journey from happy childhood to the depths of despair and my journey rising from those depths to ultimately triumph and to once again have before me that bright future that had earlier been denied. Some parts of the book are unsettling, exposing raw nerves and fears, but there are light and laughter too. It is ultimately my success story. It is a first-hand description of what bipolar disorder is.

I write this account of my life, not for myself – after so many years of therapy I really do know who I am – but for others who suffer from the same 'Two Faces in the Mirror'.

To show them that it is possible to one day look into that mirror, and see only one person smiling back. To help others through the dark days, to help their families understand they are not alone and to hopefully ignite a spark of self-confidence and joy in any sufferers themselves. If only my family and I had known when I was 13 what we know now.

I have to thank my Mom and Dad – without them holding my hand through all those dark years my demons would never have been banished. Their support and unwavering love and belief enabled me to return to sanity.

Today the mirror only has one face – mine - and I like what I see.

CHAPTER ONE

Meeting Bipolar

"Eyes, red, angry eyes glaring at me, they had found their fate- little thirteen-year-old me! Frightened, anxious, adrenalin pumping through my veins! How could I escape him? I was trapped and fenced in by this old, mad ram, feet ready to charge. And like this mad ram, so did my bipolar illness charge into my life - uninvited. "- Cally Bassage

I think a lot of people look back on their early childhood through rose-coloured spectacles, but I am consciously looking back on mine with the analytical eye of someone about to tell a factual tale, accurate in every way; the good times, the bad times and all the in-between times.

I was blessed with a particularly happy and inspiring childhood. I was a well-balanced child, living a privileged life in a secure home with caring parents and siblings. Mom and Dad always made us children feel loved and we loved and respected them in return. I was particularly close to my Mom, she was my confidant, my closest friend – funny and affectionate.

My nickname was the Pied Piper, which I think probably indicates more than anything else who I was in those days. I was always surrounded by people – even adults were part of my social circle. I must have been utterly charming! A trait I later discovered often accompanies this disease… I was special.

I remember one afternoon sitting with my sister and some friends and telling them a story – I loved telling stories. We were sprawled about as only children can be, a whole group of us and my twin Lilla (who was a quiet reserved child) and I embarked on the tale of the Slinky Malinky Butterfly.

It's a long story, but everyone loved it – especially the end which is dark but certainly appealed to my sense of humor in those days.

I spent my time doing all the things that children do, following the latest crazes and fashions as I went along. Will I ever forget my first pair of Nike sneakers? I wore them everywhere and I thought I was so very cool. I even adopted the Nike slogan as my own, it just seemed to fit – Just Do It. That was me!

I adored school and took my lessons very seriously – homework first and then playtime. I'd head straight to my room when I arrived home in the afternoons, firmly shut the door and set about doing everything - perfectly.

My siblings would be watching TV or running around outside before I was satisfied with my work. Only then was it time to play! Academically it certainly paid off, I received excellent marks. I also loved sport, especially tennis, and this received the same kind of dedication as my academic work. I was never happier than on a Friday afternoon when I'd go to Kershaw Park tennis courts and at the tender age of 12 was picked as a member of the Pietermaritzburg tennis team. I was very competitive in sports.

There was one tragic incident in those halcyon days (which I barely remember) when I nearly drowned in a friend's swimming pool. I can't quite recall how it happened, but it was a very near thing and I was already blue in the face before being resuscitated. I sometimes think that perhaps that is when I started to become a little anxious about things (anxious to achieve at school, anxious to excel on the tennis courts). I'd nearly lost my life, but God gave me another chance, He had spared me. It wouldn't be the last time.

In retrospect maybe I was a little too keen on making sure everything was perfect, but there were many other children as keen and dedicated, nothing was amiss.

However, I did feel special and like any other child, I enjoyed it when people started calling me that to my face. Cally's special. It made me feel good and gave me even more confidence and I knew, I just simply knew, that the world was there for my taking and I was capable of achieving whatever I wanted.

Perhaps there were some early warning signs of anxiety, but they were small and over quickly.

However, with the onset of my illness, my life changed – suddenly I had no control. It was like a mad raging ram had charged into my life. It also charged into the very core of my family who felt helpless facing this new situation. A feeling of emptiness and an atmosphere that became tense and urgent. We were all oblivious to the ramifications and details; understanding professionals were few and far between in those days and it was even impossible to obtain an accurate diagnosis.

Alyssa Reyans in her book, ***Letter from a Bipolar Mother***, says:

"Bipolar robs you of that which is you. It can take from you the very core of your being and replace it with something that is completely opposite of who and what you truly are."

Because my Bipolar went untreated for so long, I spent many years looking in the mirror and seeing a person I neither recognized nor understood. Not only did Bipolar rob me of my sanity, but it robbed me of my ability to see beyond the space it dictated me to look. I no longer could tell reality from fantasy and I walked in a world no longer my own."

"What do you know about bipolar disorder" I am asked. "What do *you* know?" I want to reply, but I don't, I breathe deeply and smile. "Is that the Jekyll and Hyde thing?"

I keep a neutral expression, perhaps a little bored and, although my mind and body are on the alert, I tonelessly recount, "Some people call it manic depression. It's a brain disorder that causes extreme shifts in mood and energy. It runs in families but it can be treated." I continue to breathe deeply even if I'm not smiling anymore, but inside is a different matter; my brain and my heart are pounding out different rhythms, my hands are turning cold and the back of my neck is turning hot; my throat has gone completely dry. The one thing I know about bipolar disorder is that it's a label, a label given to crazy people.

The definition of Bipolar Disorder (previously called Manic Depression) is a physical illness which manifests as a psychological illness. It is an illness of opposites (meaning two)- the mood disorder that combines the polar opposites of depression and mania. In both mania and depression, emotional processing is disturbed and both the processing of memory and the meaning of experience are distorted. The mood swings are out of proportion to external situations. In the manic phase (often referred to as a high) some of the following can be experienced : high energy levels with hyperactivity; insomnia (which is both a symptom of mania and a cause); a strong drive to work and/or tackle unnecessary tasks; plans and ideas and racing thoughts; excessive spending; unnecessary telephone calls; extreme generosity; restless, impatient, demanding and impulsive behaviour; over-inflated self-esteem and grandiose ideas and delusions; extremely irritable and easily distracted.

In the depressive stage (or low) the following symptoms can occur: extreme loss of energy; hypersomnia (excessive sleeping); the feeling of being enveloped by a black cloud; irritable.

The person has a desire to be alone; low self-esteem and feeling worthless; feelings of guilt, obsessed by past mistakes that are blown out of proportion;

an inability to experience pleasure; unable to concentrate; no interest in anyone or anything and suicidal thoughts."

CHAPTER TWO

THE ROLLERCOASTER BEGINS

It all began when I was 13. I had been very sick with bronchitis, which was simply not improving and when I was finding it difficult to breathe my Dad rushed me to the emergency room at the Medicross Medical Centre. There is a particularly unique smell about emergency rooms; maybe it's the cleaning fluids, the medication, the urgency, I don't know; I was only 13, still a child, but that smell, is an enduring memory.

The doctor quickly diagnosed that my bronchitis had developed into pneumonia, and he gave me a large dose of antibiotics and cheerfully sent us on our way. We drove home secure in the knowledge that I was now on the road to recovery.

However, things didn't go quite according to plan. Although I had competed in the Himeville tennis tournament – coming in as runner up – I felt inexplicably nervous for some reason and suddenly became very insecure. I even told my Mom at one stage that I wanted to die. I battled to sleep and was particularly anxious when my Dad was away. I was given ***Ativan**** to calm me down help me through those days and nights.

I didn't recover my full health and when I returned to school I was given a nickname, catty teenage girls decided I was to be called 'sickling'. Those words really hurt and I can't believe how cruel people can be. I was sick for days at a time and the contempt from my healthy classmates was incredibly wounding.

Although I'd enjoyed being special, this was not the same thing at all; this was 'special' in a bad way.

I couldn't concentrate properly, I missed lessons and then had to double my work in order to catch up and I worried about absolutely everything. Who would help me? Where could I turn? Who can save me from the pain? And, where, oh where, could I hide? A complete loss of self-esteem. I had moved a long way from the Pied Piper. My world had started to crumble.

I experienced my first panic attack, but of course, at that age I didn't know what it was. All I did know is that every motion was loud, like the beating of a drum getting faster and faster. I felt cold, so very very cold and I wondered if I was dead. I felt dead, but then the tingling sensation reminded me that I was alive, but my throat was so dry that I couldn't swallow. Breathe in, breathe out, breathe in, breathe out. Eventually I was back, back to life. That was my first panic attack, there were many more to follow.

I remember one day having to perform an oral at school. I had spent a long time in preparation to be sure that I would do it all perfectly. However, the more I practised the more anxious I became. Instead of growing in confidence that I would deliver this amazing oral that would enthral my classmates and the teacher, my confidence diminished daily until, when the day arrived, it had completely evaporated. By the time I stood in front of the class, my hands were shaking and I was incapable of uttering a single word. All I could think was "Get me out of here!" and promptly burst into tears. It was horrible, it was humiliating; everyone was staring at me and I had no idea what to do. My teacher was very calm and explained that this sort of thing happens to a lot of people and that I could perform my oral to her privately.

Suddenly the sun was shining again, I would be able to deliver my well-planned and erudite oral to my teacher in private.

I felt like a princess. Special. I was not normal! I was not like everyone else! The fear and the guilt and the condemnation of these feelings only made matters worse.

A couselling psychologist with an interest in child psychology - Floss Mitchell, entered my life. She was like the buoy that life-savers use to rescue people from the sea. Yes! She was a life-saver!

I was very nervous about meeting her for the first time, but I understood that my situation needed some external intervention. However, Floss was warm and approachable and had a motherly protective manner. I found I could confide in her, tell her all the worries that were causing a little 13-year-old such grief. Floss took me seriously and she listened to everything I said. It was the beginning of a long journey together.

It was about that time that a friend had a freak accident during a rugby match. The young fit healthy man had his future changed in one split second when he became paralysed. Floss explained that what was happening to me was similar in that both our futures had been irrevocably altered by one small event.

I met with Floss once a week at her rooms in Pietermaritzburg where she taught me various relaxation exercises to help me combat stress at school, especially those frightening panic attacks which had become more frequent and terrifying. One exercise, in particular, made a big impact and I still use it to this day. It is a visualisation exercise and Floss would talk me through it in her calm voice.

" Imagine you are this heavy beaded necklace that has been dropped in the big ocean, there is stillness and silence all around as the necklace descends lower and lower to the bottom of the ocean, it gets darker and darker and silence, utter silence, deepness of the ocean, and then it falls and rests at the ground on the bottom of the ocean, silence!"

Floss taught me to also do deep breathing where the air meets my diaphragm in the bottom of my belly and whenever I felt the start of agonising panic I was trained to take a moment and do this deep breathing. The most amazing thing is that it worked (for a while at least).

However, I did need more professional help. The antibiotic injection that had been administered to me for my pneumonia, (before the onset of the anxiety and depression) was in all likelihood still in my system and, as is the habit of antibiotics, played havoc with my small body. I went to see a local Pietermaritzburg psychiatrist, Dr Lund. Many more psychiatrists would follow over the years, but Dr Lund was my first.

I became very fond of Dr Lund. At that time my panic attacks were the main issue and he thought of various ways in which he could help, but the attacks were escalating and had progressed into dark depressions, rather like how cancer spreads from Stage 1 to Stage 4, suffocating every cell in the body.

My anxiety had the effect of depleting the serotonin in my body and as a result, I was experiencing nightmarish hallucinations. I felt desperately alone and was absolutely terrified. I was unhealthy, skin and bone and although I didn't consciously think of it at the time, I was fighting the monumental battle for my sanity.

I was prescribed the tranquiliser *Ativan*, to relax me in anxious times. I was also medicated with various other anti-depressants and mood stabilizers, but at the end of the day despite all the medication, I was still not well. What on earth was wrong with me? Three weeks of a month I'd be on a roller-coaster of ups and downs. My parents became desperate. I was going through puberty so perhaps I had a hormonal imbalance? Hopefully I paid a visit to an endocronologist, but of course, nothing helped in the end, absolutely nothing. Despite being surrounded by a loving family, I felt I was completely and utterly alone and I was very very frightened.

As a perfectionist and high-achiever always trying to excel, it's hardly any wonder that the wheels came off – from a very fast car as well! Dr Lund, as my psychiatrist, was perplexed and we still had been unable to find a working solution.

My parents were also becoming increasingly desperate to find a solution as I was not getting better, I was getting worse. Panic and darkness became my constant companions accompanied by strange obscure and maddening thoughts. I would watch my parents at night as they slept soundly and all I wanted was to be able to gently fall asleep beside them. My main ambition at the time was to return to normality – back to the successful happy little girl I had been. "I just want to be normal". You will see this theme echoed time and time again during the course of this book.

An extact from my mom's diary: 21 April 1996

"Woke up at 12pm, came to our room. Slept 3am. Started anxiety. Motions on and off needed reassurance all the time. Bathed 5.30am. Had herbalife drink (protein drink).

About 11am she started coming right and told me that she was feeling more normal. Told me that orals were not going to be forced on her. She said after her working through with Floss she may be ready to give orals. At 6pm gave Cal a tofranil. Still silent sleep. No supper"

It is evident that I found school very stressful, both internally and externally.

Things that were possible to control, ie: when it was time to do my homework were bearable, but the things over which I had no control, (relationships, friendships, teenage pressures and the general environment), were just too much for me.

Teenagers always find life tough at some point – they wouldn't be teenagers if they didn't and it is perhaps one of the most challenging times in any one's life. Those teenage years for me, a chemically unbalanced girl, were particularly tough. I was missing so much school and had become a constant worry to my family. How very hard it must have been for them. Reading through my Moms diary I see one day is good, another day bad, I was leading them on a similar up and down path as my own. I was on **Tofranil** and sleeping tablets – even on holiday in the Kruger Park.

My anxiety and delusions simply would not keep away and one evening my Mom had to phone Dr Lund whom we met at Greys Hospital. I was convinced I was a male and nothing could persuade me otherwise. I didn't want to go to the hospital, I didn't want to be admitted, but I was over-ruled and given a calming injection.

I didn't know what on earth was happening to me. "I just want to be normal", I told my Mom.

Floss, quietly weeping, was there, as neither she, nor my mom, nor my dad, nor it seemed anyone else, knew exactly what was wrong with me.

We all felt completely helpless.

And then my mom sang a lullaby, " I will never let you go, never let you go, because I love you, because I love you, I will never let you go, never let you go because I love you, little girl." I fell into a deep sleep. I was so loved, my mom loved me so much and that is all I needed to know and feel.

I isolated myself from everyone in the hospital, I refused further medication, became obstructive and stubborn and at times even violent. I was very highly medicated and disorientated. All I wanted to do was go home.

When I was discharged it was to a strict regime that had been discussed with Dr Lund. A lot of encouragement, but no medication. I'd lost 5kg during that short stay in hospital and was physically frail; I couldn't even walk all the way around the garden. My Mom prayed with all her might, "I pray she has a better day tomorrow, please Jesus, help us to help her."

Tomorrow, however, was not a better day. I paged through old Christmas and birthday cards and decided that the world was a horrible place. I wanted to escape and one day I set off to do just that. I climbed over the gate and ran helter-skelter down the road, luckily someone who knew me saw me and stopped me, they carried me back home.

School had become completely different. I was no longer the high achiever, I was 'the Sickling'.

The teachers were understanding and incredibly patient and compassionate and obviously never asked me to do orals ever again, but I had missed so many days and my close friends had drifted away leaving me isolated. Life seemed pointless.

One day at school I took a handful of *Ativan*. I remember looking at the pills as they rested gently in my hand before I swallowed them all before quietly returning to class. I was knocked out pretty quickly and the shocked teacher instantly called my mom. It was this attempted suicide which really brought home to my parents that I was NOT getting better, I was becoming worse, I was going downhill. My parents were desperate, no one really knew what to do.

CHAPTER THREE

LOOKING FOR SOLUTIONS

I was sixteen. It had been three years since I became ill, three long disruptive and painful years, not only for me but for my family.

Life had its normal times, sometimes for weeks on end and during one of those normal times I fell in love as only a 16-year-old can – madly and completely (no pun intended). James (not his real name) was my first real boyfriend. At the advanced age of 19 he was, as far as I was concerned, the most handsome boy in the world, the funniest and the smartest and I absolutely adored him. It was simple, I loved him and he loved me.

We were passionately in love and spent much time kissing and cuddling and just being with each other. To me it was like a dream, it was like the movies – I was his princess and he was my prince. However, my illness was still there and I wasn't completely stable and one day, for no rhyme or reason, I sent him a blistering email terminating our relationship. When I returned to sanity and realised what I had done, I was completely devastated and tried to explain to James, but without the benefit of a proper diagnosis of my problem I floundered in my explanation. James, who had been hurt and confused by my rejection sadly never did understand, but perhaps in retrospect, it was for the best and he did not have to share my madness.

As a family we all placed our hope in doctors, in modern medicine, in institutions – this is what we all clung to.

We heard that Tara Psychiatric Hospital in Johannesburg specialized in anorexia and bipolar with great success. We thought we'd found the solution. Was Tara going to be our breakthrough – our hope for the future?

Mom and I packed the car and drove up to Johannesburg – anxious, but very hopeful that the doctors would be able to provide a proper diagnosis as to my problem. I was sick most of the time. Actually, I often thought I was Jesus and invincible – I was like God and soared with the eagles. I even went around to friends and families to convince them they were all my chosen disciples – almost succeeding in some cases! I was very mystical and attractive and my goodness, how adventurous I was! I was King Arthur's beloved queen and we rode side-by-side to Camelot.

Tara was a hospital that specialized in the diagnosis of bipolar, but we were warned that it could take months before reaching an accurate diagnosis.

On arrival, I was taken by surprise at the warmth of Tara – not cold and clinical which is the first thought that comes to mind when people mention a Psychiatric Hospital. It had a homely feel about it and I instantly felt comfortable despite being in a manic state. It was to be my home for the next six months.

The first doctor to see me at Tara was Dr Tibby Chizmadia. Dr Chizmadia was a kind, friendly man and I felt instinctively that he could be trusted, so I didn't fear the terms that were given for me to be admitted. My parents seemed happier and very hopeful and I believed I would receive the best care possible and by God's grace soon be on my way to good health. There was a long journey ahead, I knew that, but it was a journey to be undertaken if I was ever to have any kind of meaningful life.

As I was under 18 I was admitted to the children's ward where there were other teenage girls.

They suffered from all sorts of problems ranging from suicidal and aggressive issues to anxiety – I was one of them. The first friend I made was Jessica and we shared a bunk bed. Jessica adored Leonardo di Caprio and had a poster of him hanging on the wall.

Truly, Madly, Deeper, a song by Savage Garden was often played from her walkie-talkie. A part of me realised that I was institutionalized, I was a patient at a psychiatric hospital – I was stigmatized – but I didn't care what people back at home might be thinking as Tara had become my new home. I felt safe and quickly became accustomed to the people with all their varying forms of mental imbalance. These people became my friends, they were fun and they were good company.

My companions were not inmates of a jail, but precious special people who had a need to reclaim their sanity, just like me. I was there to find relief from my own madness, to escape the racing thoughts, the lightning bolts of senseless energy, the chemicals going haywire in my head.

Dr Chizmadia was wonderful – actually at one stage I developed a childlike crush on him – and I admired him enormously for his patience and understanding, as well as his humour, much needed in his line of work. A lot of time was spent monitoring and assessing me; the habits and behaviour in my manic state were undeniably traits of bipolar disease, although at that point I had not experienced the swing-high swing-low effect. I was unmistakably high and manic and after three months of observation I was formally diagnosed with bipolar disorder.

Bipolar - the name that is given to crazy people, to those who belong in the funny farm and now it seemed I was one of them.

At that stage, I was actually unaware of the stigma attached to mental illness and I was too young and naive to even give a damn, I was just convinced and happy that having received a proper diagnosis, I was on the road to recovery. My parent's relief was tangible – here it was, finally, hope! Hope that their bright, pretty little girl would be returned to them and to her life.

The last couple of years had taken a huge toll on the family and being presented with the diagnosis and a plan of moving forward can only be described as wonderful in the true sense of the word.

Life at Tara was good – even the food was fantastic and I often queued up for seconds.

I was there during a hot summer and under the supervision of a psychiatric nurse, we would often swim in the pool. There were even two rugby fields on the grounds and my family brought me various sports equipment so that I could practice my skills – a soccer ball, a golf club.

My mom stayed with family members that lived in Jo'burg and visited me nearly every day, initially even helping me bathe and shaving my legs – most important to a teenager and we weren't allowed our own razors for obvious reasons. Mom would always sing her special lullaby, "I will never let you go, never let you go, never let you go. Why? Because I love my little girl." It was so reassuring and led me eventually back to becoming the Cally everyone knew and loved.

There was a small school at Tara and I relished being back in the classroom again.

I was still that high achiever and despite missing almost half my school years up to 16 I still passed really well. I was still a brilliant child! Special!

Tara was a Godsend – perhaps that is why the sunsets were so beautiful.

I would tackle tasks with diligence at Occupational Therapy. I became well behaved, the manic phase easing its way out. Medicated with lithium, a drug commonly used to stabilize the manic phases of bipolar, I was becoming calmer. Tara was for me a home from home, beautiful and, most importantly, a hopeful place.

After six months it was time to go home. I had been diagnosed, prescribed medicine that worked and normal life awaited me. However, I had not paid much attention to the stigma of the label and the severity of that label cannot be underestimated. I had a mental condition, a dark and misunderstood condition. I was told that one in ten people have bipolar and 30% not only attempt, but succeed in committing suicide.

This added a further dimension to the problem as it suddenly became a life-threatening disease as well. I tried not to think about it at the time, it was too enormous. There was and always will be the stigma, from which I would learn I could not escape. I was bipolar. I have bipolar. I am who I am. I am Cally. I am and always will be Cally.

Swing high, swing low, elevated moods, depressing moods – these characterise my illness, but it is with joy that I understand there is always hope.

CHAPTER FOUR

TO AND FRO

Back home! Everything should have felt familiar and comforting, but I felt distanced and the familiar had become unfamiliar and I was filled with a sense of deep unease. I reminded myself to take one day at a time. I took my first bubble-bath in what seemed like years and years – the sense of freedom (unsupervised) was like unwrapping an unexpected gift. Slowly I embraced the new Cally and found myself getting a little stronger, a little more confident, day by day. The medication had taken effect; there were no more highs or lows. I felt normal! Of course, who knows what normal means? All I knew was that I was no longer sick in the head, maddened by the psychotic symptoms of bipolar illness and my life was returning. However, in the back of my mind was the ever-recurring question – how long would this last?

I returned to school full of hope. It was not a good experience as although I had attended lessons at Tara they had not kept pace with St. Johns. Academically I was able to cope and although I was only there for half of the school year I took the lessons in my stride and passed Grade 10. However, fitting back into the social network was the problem, the big disappointment.

My peers seemed vague in their interactions with me and I found myself feeling very detached. My twin tried to include me with her friends, but I felt like the constant outsider and bore the brunt of still being referred to as "the Sickling".

It was horribly unfair, but of course by that time I had realised that life is not fair and can be very cruel.

Grade 11 quickly followed but remains a blur in my memory as I sank into deep depressions. These depressions were not the same as my previous ones where I would hallucinate and suffer psychotic nightmares. It seemed as if I was living my worst nightmare every day. Occasionally I would experience bipolar highs where I would become incredibly creative, writing and art, but the swing-high-swing-low effect created extreme exhaustion and I eventually came to a complete standstill and needed to go back to Tara.

However, I was now 18 and was admitted to the adult ward (quite different from the homely children's ward) and found myself in a tiny cell with one small window and just a mattress on the floor. It felt as if I was a criminal, but at the time I was so exhausted that I fell into a deep sedated sleep. Mom lovingly kept watching by my side. I can only imagine how helpless she must have felt – all our hopes and fears in the hands of the doctors and praying for Divine intervention. Days of sleep turned slowly into weeks.

The adult ward was not a nice place to be. The people really were all crazy, schizophrenics, depressants and bipolar – and I was one of them! I slept on that mattress on the floor and the only real comfort was being allowed to wear my own clothes after my mother had obtained formal permission. Together with my own clothes and my Moms lovely blanket I derived some small comfort, well away from the world in which I found myself.

I was trapped in that cell and even when I needed to relieve myself, no one answered my call. I can remember the warmth of my urine as it slid down my legs.

I became desperate to be rescued – even if only being given the privilege of being able to go to the bathroom when I needed to.

I found a friend there – Terrence – who brought me some comfort and much strength. He wore t-shirts emblazoned with smiley faces and at heart was the ultimate perfectionist. He was very fond of me in that Big Brother way. Terrence loved his music and would often pace up and down the corridor plugged into his favourite song and sometimes he would let me listen too. I regret to this day not keeping in contact with him once I left Tara.

Once we were asked to line up like the military and were walked down to the Rugby field where we discovered it was our Sports Day. There was volleyball, netball, basketball, soccer, tennis and swimming on the programme. Participation was optional and initially, I was not keen, but I did enjoy a good game of volleyball. I imagine it was a fun way to introduce us patients to strenuous exercise to increase our wellbeing with natural dopamine (fondly known as the happy hormone and produced naturally by the body during exercise).

So the days passed. I had been there for four months; starting with flying high in the stratosphere and furiously crashing down, hiding like a mole deep underground. However, the medication, particularly lithium, gradually stabilised my moods. Thank you Dr Chizmadia – or was it Divine Intervention?

CHAPTER FIVE

HIDDEN GIFTS & DEEP DESPAIR

Manic episodes often stimulate creativity and during this period intelligent and beautiful writings are done; artistic masterpieces are created as the brilliance of the mind is unleashed. Michael Angelo and the Sistine Chapel spring to mind and there is evidence that Leonardo Da Vinci was also bipolar. Others include Abraham Lincoln, Beethoven, Mozart, Tchaikovsky, Mark Twain, Winston Churchill – the list goes on.

In one of my manic episodes, I sat and wrote my story – I called it The Memoirs of a Bipolar sufferer. I include it here, uncut, unedited and in its original form. It was where I was, at that particular time.

Here is an extract from my draft book - Memoirs of a bipolar sufferer

I sit with my distressed parents, unannounced in the waiting room, the room which is so familiar to me. The receptionist says that the doctor is ready to see me. Amidst the chaos in my mind, I understand the importance of the situation. The doctor stares at me and asks me how I am feeling. There was a sight of desperation on both my mom and dad's face; their last hope was left in the hands of the doctor. I could hear dogs barking and cars driving past in the distance. All I wanted was to go home. But staring at the doctor I knew this was my fate, another inclusion to yet another psychiatric hospital. This is the story of my life.

The nurse tells me that I can wear my own casual clothes instead of wearing a hospital uniform. I remember being relieved at least I would not be looking like a wanted criminal. Amongst the patients at Townhill Hospital there were people with many different mental conditions. The hospital lived up to its stigmatic reputation as being a place for crazy people, people who have lost the plot, people who belong in the "funny" farm and I was one of them.

I remember the wrought iron framed beds that made a noise every time I turned around in my sleep. I avoided as much as possible not to eat any of the food. The food served was a mere attempt at what you called food. Mom and Dad were consistent in bringing me lunch and supper every day which was something that I looked forward to.

I was rudely awakened by the matron when she said that it was time for showering. Her stern voice motivated me to get out of bed in a hurry. She was a horrid lady who over the years had been overworked and had resolved to become a grumpy and cynical woman. I was not surprised to learn that I was not the only one who feared her.

Standing in a row, completely naked. I could feel our skins rubbing against each other.

We were homed in like sheep being lined up for dipping at least that is what it felt like. There was a frail, bare breasted woman who after all her suffering stood naked in front of me. We were shown no respect irrespective of age. This reminded me of the film, "Schindlers List," where the Jewish Refugees were forced to huddle together in the shower with little remorse from the German army. We are now living in the twenty-first century this kind of behaviour should not be allowed.

I remember getting my body wet while waiting to use the shared soap. Were we animals? Just because we had lost touch of reality did it mean that we had no right to be treated like people? We already felt undignified, why make it worse?

It all began at the youthful age of thirteen. So young. Little did I know then that this was the beginning of my journey of pain. My teenage years, my high school days are of a blurred image with only momentary glimpses of sunlight in between.

I began having hallucinations. Hallucinations that belong in your worst nightmare! I was having a shower and instead of water coming out-blood did! I would also frequently get visits from an evil clown.

There were phone calls from people all over the world sharing their concerns. My family were very distressed, there was no end to my pain. My bad state would occur for when only a week in the month I would be feeling normal. In that week I would try and catch up on missed school work and as I was a high achiever missed school work added to more stress. I was also battling to maintain my friendships at school.

I was usually seen as the sporty extrovert but had resolved to become shy and withdrawn. The word desperate does not give justice to the pain I was feeling. I was trapped and could not see any other way out. I began plotting my suicide. I stopped thinking about the selfishness of the act, about how it would destroy my family, I didn't care, I wanted to die more than anything. I remember the family were sitting watching television in the lounge and I silently went to the medicine box in my parents' bedroom and took all the pills and emptied them onto the bed.

I then swallowed all my prescribed medicine and all the other pills I then closed my eyes and went to bed hoping never to wake up.

But I woke up from that dreary sleep, thinking that I was in Heaven, but I was sick again and hell loomed over me. Why God? I wanted to shout and scream, but I didn't, I was too weak. Too much pain...I wanted to die again.

The cross is a scary place to live - not to die. It is where the light is found but also where my pain and suffering began again. Jesus lover of my soul? I questioned God, even more pain. I look to the cross, He alone is my rock, my strength, without Him I am nothing. Am I higher than the living God? Why so much pain? Why so much suffering? And why so much forgiveness? I love you, God, more and less each day. God spoke and I listened. Where to run to? Where to hide? I am waiting for you.

The intensity of knowing one's pain is entering into that darkest place within one's soul. Seldom dare to go there but I believe that is where one comes to the essence of who you are when you can look beneath the surface and go deeper and stop for a moment and look within yourself. Throughout my pain and suffering I have learnt that joy and peace really start when you seek your own heart. When you can come before yourself and almost take your heart out of your chest to the realization that life is not much about popularity or fame or even existence, it's about knowing who you are.

It's about being humble, not proud and walking a life of servitude always knowing your heart before it even beats and knowing your failures and learning from them. Walking in forgiveness always knowing that your heart and mind and soul are well.

Some people say, "Stop and smell the roses," but I say stop and take a breath and look within you will be surprised to find that you are surrounded with strength and amazing beauty!

Don't be afraid to cry because when you cry you are most alive that is when God's spirit is moving within you, touching you with His healing.

I have cried and laughed. My joys have been as vast as my sorrows. The journey of a bipolar sufferer is not an easy one. I have known the intensities of a mixture of colourful emotions from love to despair and then wonderful euphoria. I've known that to love in ecstasy is like running naked on a freezing night through an open field, to love is to feel the richness of a good coffee or to see a child smile for the first time. I was in love, love with places, people and energy.

The vibe of the city, the lights all around me. At night people moving, cars buzzing around. During the day, movement, ongoing movement. Yes I was in love? Should I stay or should I go? Stop the red light said! But I couldn't dare tell anyone, but was I in love? All I could think of was possibilities, objects, things, even opportunities! For me? Little insignificant me? The world my oyster! Johannesburg smelt like a fresh Spring morning, like rain after a hot day. I was addicted to energy. Completely addicted.

I was oblivious to the warning signs, the dreaded signs that cry out as I was in euphoria and didn't want to stop. It just felt too good. Mad spending sprees or rather giving away of little I had. Talking too much and at rapid speeds, high expectations and illusions of self. To die to Christ and to give to mankind, what was I thinking? Was I playing God? Or was I just merely crazy? Tara psychiatric hospital was a constant thought as I drove past the area.

But soon I'd be taken back, back to reality to the boring mundaneness of life. Depression penetrating glass cutting through my veins and into my being, poisoning and intoxicating me. Help someone!

But all the rats did was hide under the rubble and eat away at the perfectly moulded and happy life of mine. Yet my heart still beat diastolic and systolic beats in my chest, beats rhythmic pulsating beats, beats to the city life yet I was dead, I had finished the race inside, "Way out! Cooked! Fried! Crazy! Or maybe even just maybe normal?

I doubt it. Far from normal was what I was. Manic and flitting higher, higher above the cotton wool clouds above the aeroplane wings, high, soaring high above everything. Is this what heaven feels like? So good like sweets and candy floss! Crash! Bang! Collapsed like a dead heap of cement.

Dead and heavy, not knowing where to run, too anxious inside. Help! Stop the shouting inside, can anyone hear me or are you all deaf? Deaf and dumb, numbed by the intoxicating poisons of the chemicals of the little happy packet of smarties that slide down the oesophagus into the stomach of my belly every morning and night- anti-depressants, mood stabilizers, tranquilizers, anti-psychotics. Zombie! I am a living zombie! But my heart still pulsating to the beat of the ongoing madness.

Thoughts everywhere, confusion controlling my mind, non-nonsensical words, little boys and girls shouting, laughing, swimming up and down the lanes, even railway tracks on white teeth, a smile, a shudder, "don't look at me!" The darkness of the under level parking bay, darkness all around. I park my car huddled between the pillars, the security guard asks me if I know my way. He's drunk! Run! I think to myself, he could rape me!

My head is spinning. I look upstairs to climb, he is behind me! God save me. Depression sits in, I try but I can't. Nothing. Emptiness. Yet my heart still beats in my chest.

Depression, how can I explain to you? Dark underworld of pitifulness, nothing, black, grey, morbid fascinations, death and horror. All by myself, totally alone, lonely. No God, no faith, faithless.

Little girls crying and dogs barking in the distance and worst of all broken relationships, unmended hearts. Pain. Too much sorrow and too much pain. Just another day. Just live one more day.

And then as soon as it began it ended.

Sunlight, hope and a future! Yesterday compared with today, a million miles apart! The light has been switched on! No more frowning but a radiant smile! I picked up the shattered pieces of my relationships and glued them together. I spoke to him, the undaunted, unblemished one and he understood. Relief, peace and unity.

God save me from another bipolar episode! Yet mostly inevitable. I am who I am between the highs and lows and that is where I find my hope and reality and sanity. I cling to what I know which is my faith and let it carry me through all the badness. The dimensions of the realities in my mind and the obscurities of the unforgettable thoughts, all the intensity, colours, visions and feelings of euphoric ecstasy! Highs, way above, God-like and living to the ultimate. What it means to have bipolar!

Such mixed emotions of ideas and feelings. After all it is bipolar the dreaded disease, the brilliant disease!

Normality is a rare word for a bipolar sufferer yet that is what I feel now. There is always hope amidst the chaos and confusion. I have despaired yet been reminded to just live another day that tomorrow might be the turning point.

My hope for you the reader is to live another day, madness has no power, it is the alluring cowardliness of the thoughts one has yet you have the power to rise and to live.

CHAPTER SIX

HIGHS & HALLUCINATIONS

The time at Tara in the adult ward, despite being terrifying, had served its purpose. Once again I was stable and back home in Pietermaritzburg and facing the normal challenges of everyday life. I was doing pretty well and having missed so much school was home-schooling with five other scholars. There was freedom! There was fun! I developed some deep friendships with my fellow homeschoolers, particularly a boy called Jeffrey (not his real name); drawn together by our Christianity and good conversation Jeffrey remains a good friend to this day. Homeschool was a good change for me and I was very fond of our teacher (though I imagine today her love of cigarettes and the fact that most of her students also smoked would be frowned upon).

I changed my subjects that year from the more 'arty' package I had originally selected at St. Johns, to Business Economics, Economics, Criminology, Maths, English and Afrikaans. I loved these new subjects, especially criminology where I learnt about the motives and minds of criminals – I was fascinated. I often wonder if that fascination did not stem from feelings I had experienced in the past when I had felt like a criminal whilst in Town Hill or Tara. Somehow I felt I could relate.

Bipolar episodes seemed a long way away and I was happy. But, nothing lasts forever and unbeknown to me at the time, another episode was approaching and before I knew it there I was again - surrounded by darkness and desperately seeking a place to hide.

I was taken to Entabeni Hospital (in Durban), arriving on a manic high convinced I was Jesus and entirely capable of performing countless miracles (and of course walk upon water). I instantly recruited the other patients in the ward as my disciples and, although I was actually parading up and down on a well-manicured lawn, I KNEW beyond a shadow of a doubt, that I was walking on water!

At Entabeni, everyone was my friend – I was the Holy Man! I was the Holy Man with a cigarette! I might have been able to resist the temptation from my home-schooling teacher, but this time I gave in and cigarettes became my friends as well. Mom didn't leave me any money as she disapproved of smoking and knew I'd buy cigarettes not snacks if she did so. I became a bargainer with my fellow patients – my pudding for your cigarette! There was an old lady who smoked flavoured cigarettes all the way from England, these were my favourite, very long and very graceful, just like my gran would have smoked in her day.

One day a group of black ladies dressed in white paid a visit to the opposite ward and I heard the familiar sound of hymns and prayer. I went and took a little look and they invited me to join them. Thankfully at that stage I no longer thought I was Jesus I think I would have caused quite a stir had I marched in there ready to perform miracles! Dr Salduker had managed to find the right medication to lead me from my psychosis.

Even though I wasn't completely sane I think I was a comfort to some of the other patients. One lady, in particular, was so full of pain and anxiety, distressed beyond measure at being there but realizing she had no other option.

I repeatedly reassured her that everything was going to be OK in the end, ECT therapy was painless and would soon be over.

I looked over her small frame and could see the ECT room – a cold and unwelcoming place. I had received ECT therapy between the ages of 13 and 16 and although initially, the results had seemed positive, they did not last long. I could not tell this poor panicked soul any of this, perhaps her results would be more long-lasting than my own. Perhaps they would take her out of clinical depression. Who knows?

My memories of Entabeni definitely fall into the category of crazy – maybe that's because I WAS crazy at the time. For example, I hated Group Therapy – they wouldn't let me tap my feet up and down, they called it 'restless syndrome'. I also became a chain smoker – cigarettes were my only joy. I only wished for the day when I could go home, to Mom, Dad and my siblings.

The days seemed to last forever and although Mom and Dad phoned me daily, I felt so far away from them. When I think of those times I know beyond a shadow of a doubt that their love and support was the anchor of my healing. Their sacrifice and commitment and unconditional love saw me through.

CHAPTER SEVEN

MISSING PIECES

One of the greatest tragedies of bipolar illness is the way it steals so much of one's life. Months and weeks are lost, gone forever. I was never consistently well in my 20s and so unable to pursue a university degree, bipolar was always in the way. In those broken years, I managed a Diploma in Natural Health and Holistic Massage, although the course took an extra year to complete. I thoroughly enjoyed the massage and very quickly I became the family masseuse. I was inspired to think of the future and planned to open my own Holistic Massage salon.

The insidious tentacles of bipolar have far-reaching effects, just as soon as I had laid my plans, they were thwarted. The highs and lows and the ever-moving unquantifiable graph of going up and down are invisible at times – the line between sanity and insanity is grey and insubstantial, but of indelible ink. Once I drove to Cape Town in my 'Bumble Bee', (my little canary yellow golf). No one had the faintest idea that I was borderline manic. By the time I arrived in the Cape and was welcomed into the home of my Moms best friend I was, to all intents and purposes, completely insane. My hosts had no idea of what was going on, or how to help me and phoned my parents, to tell them I was acting 'very strangely'. Dad was on the next flight to Cape Town! I was having another bipolar episode and he wrapped me in a blanket, put me on the backseat of Bumblebee and quietly drove me home. I was depleted, desperate. How wonderful to feel powerful, to believe oneself to be invincible, but always, deep inside, to know the dangers that lie within.

That is what often led me to seek the safety of my beloved Bumble Bee. Driving one day I ran out of petrol – it was dark and I was on a mountain road, the wind howling and I was definitely in a manic frame of mind. Anything could have happened, but my unusual behaviour had been noted by a nearby restaurant owner who phoned my brother.

Another time I hit Jo'burg. I was brilliant and had secured a massage job and after only a few days my boss offered me a managerial position. I was over the moon – success was there, within my hands. Jo'burg was so full of hope and energy and how I loved those bright lights. I really felt the world was my oyster, happiness and normality, a future full of boundless opportunity. Too bad it didn't last. That was the pattern of my existence, it ended as quickly as it started and I was struck down with another bipolar episode.

The common denominator of most psychiatric illness is how their devastating episodes robs the sufferer of time, denying them the joys (and challenges) of life. The more insidious and equally devastating fact is that it also robs those that love you, they also suffer and lose time whilst clinging desperately to hope that the chaos and pain will come to an end. My youth, my teenage years and my 20s were like a plague of locusts gluttonously destroying every living thing in their way.

And how perplexing is bipolar! It is a colourful maverick of a disease, evoking creativity and generosity and feelings of grandeur. But then it turns to darkness and stagnation, dragging it's sufferer down to complete mental paralysis.

Sometimes it can be beautiful, always intriguing, but dangerous enough to wipe out your life in an instant. I knew from early on that these feelings of euphoria would not last, but whilst experiencing them I had no clue.

The nurses however knew and carefully kept me in a guarded lock-up. There was that mattress on the floor again! At the time I didn't care, I had no idea of my predicament and was cheerfully soaring high above the clouds. Deep inside though, I knew it would only be a matter of time before I would plummet.

The Mirror has Two Faces

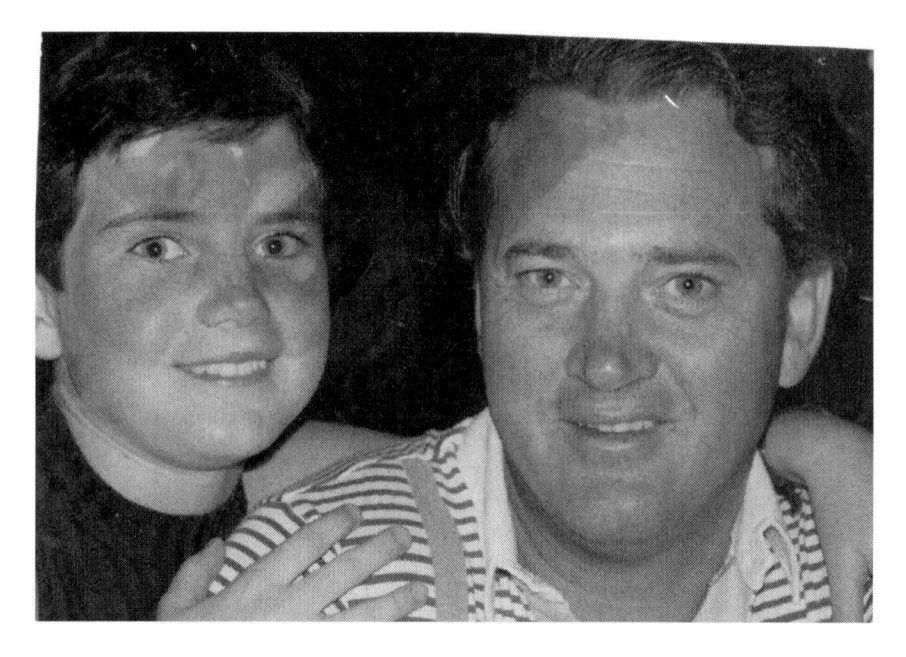

Me (left) and my Dad Jack (right) during my early years when everything was still carefree and normal.
Below : The grounds at Tara Psychiatric Hospital in Johannesburg, here I was finally diagnosed and given treatment.

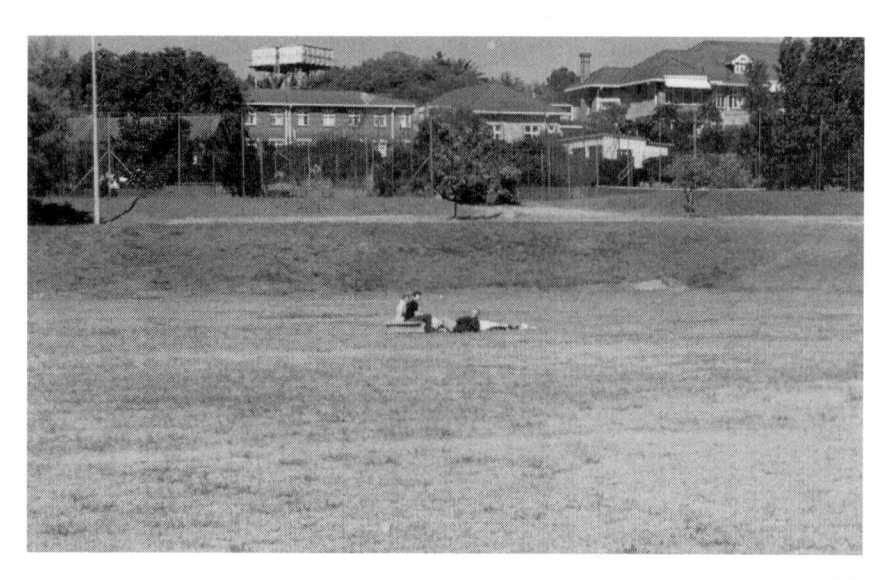

The Mirror has Two Faces

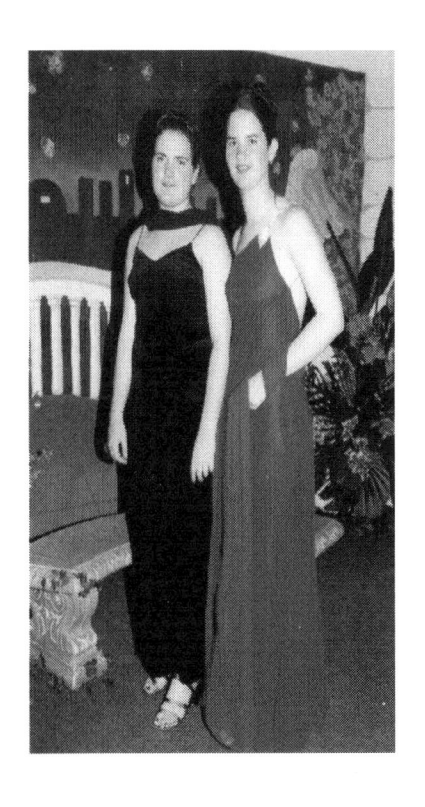

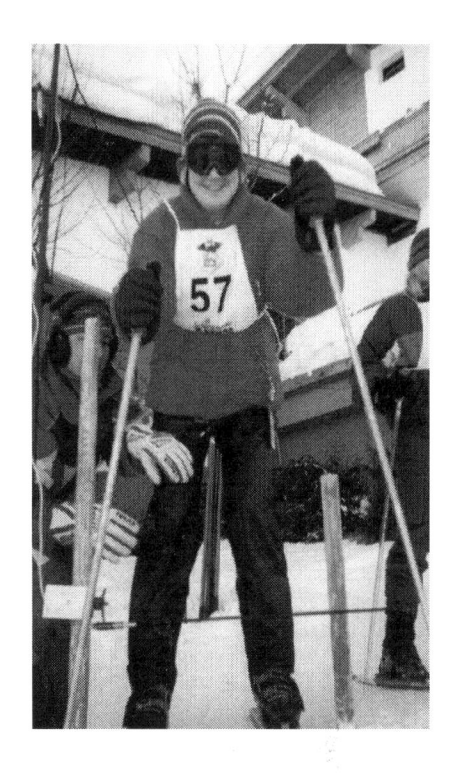

Left:
Me and my twin sister Lilla (in red) ready for our matric dance.

Right:
This was me on our overseas ski-ing holiday. I was in a manic phase and thought I could do anything. I was invincible.

The Mirror has Two Faces

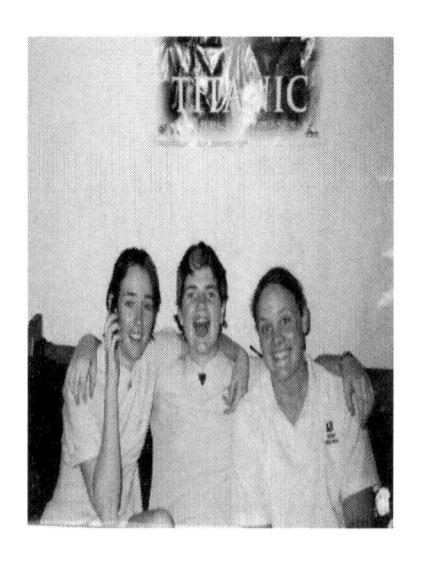

Left:

Me and two friends from St John's College in Pietermaritzburg where I went to school. When I became ill it was very hard to cope with the pressures of school.

Below:

Mom, Bridget, Me and Lilla during an overseas trip

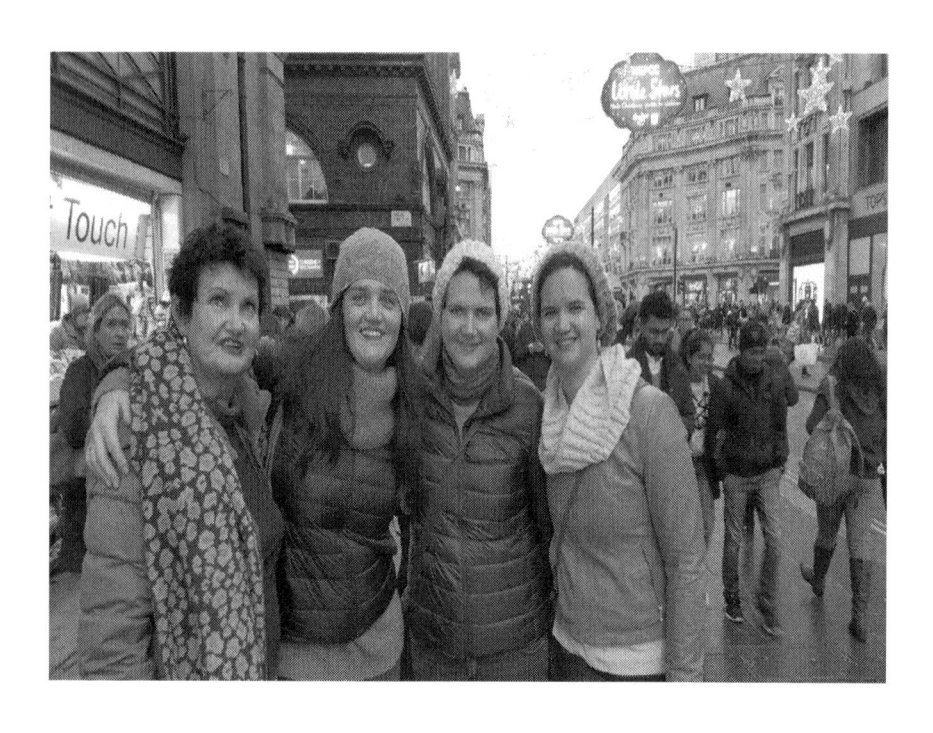

44

The Mirror has Two Faces

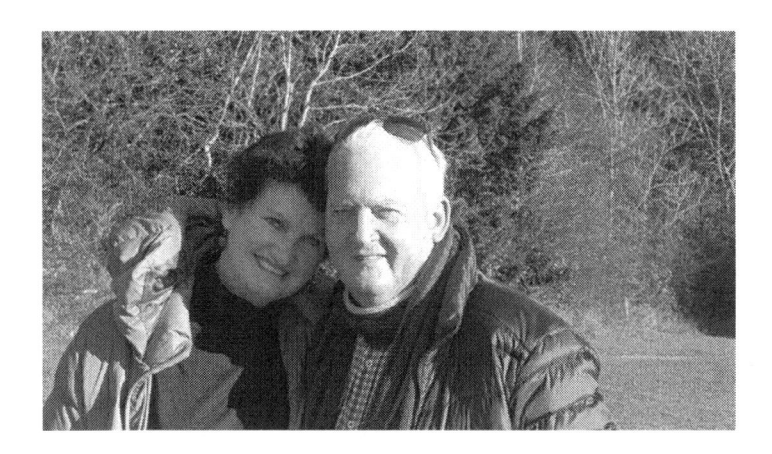

Above: Sue Bassage (Mom) and Jack Bassage (Dad) their love and support got me through some very dark times and their faith in my recovery never wavered.

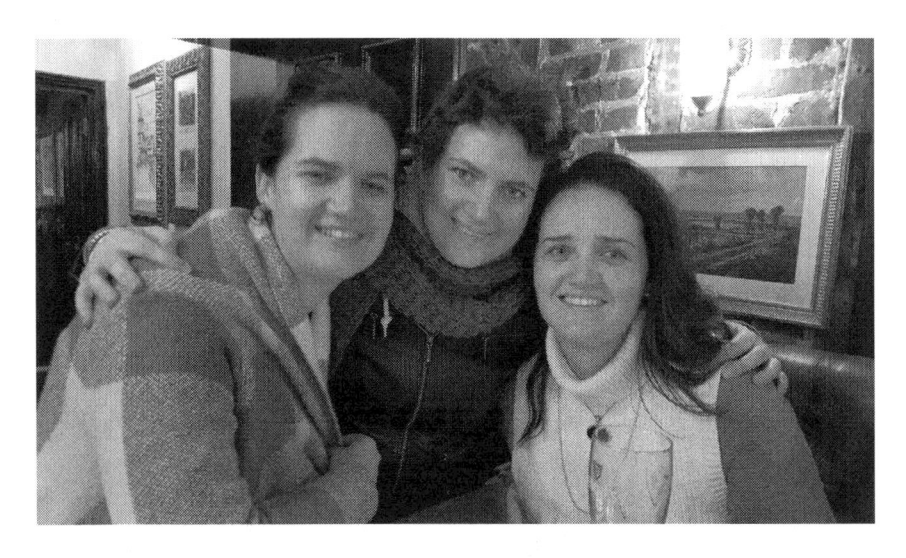

Above: Sister love – being part of twins is difficult as people invariably compare you, but my illness made me feel miles behind my sister Lilla (left). But her and my younger sister Bridget (right) were always kind and supportive.

The Mirror has Two Faces

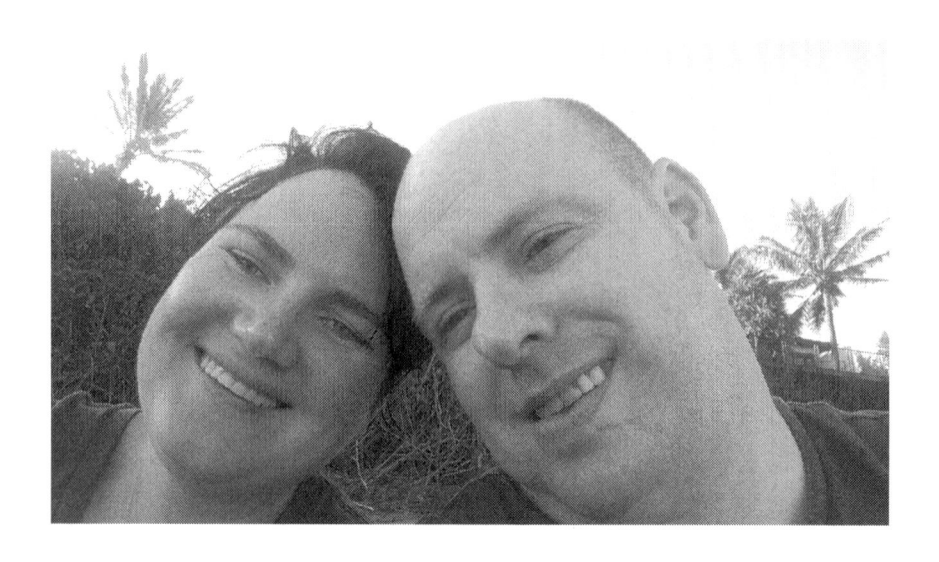

Above: Finding love has been a great way to feel normal. Greg (right) is one of the most compassionate and understanding people in my life.

Below: My family have sacrificed a lot and learnt a lot from my struggle with bipolar disorder. My brother Derrin (far left) today has much more empathy and understanding for others who are dealing with mental illness.

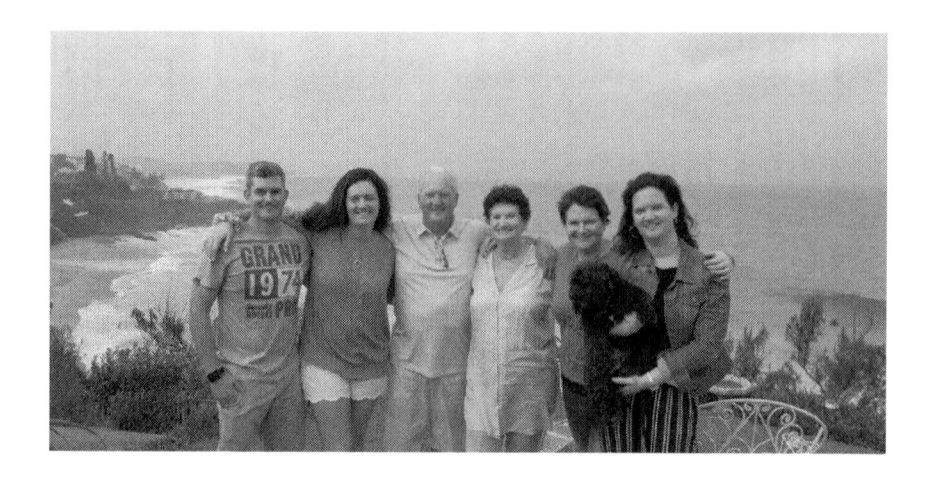

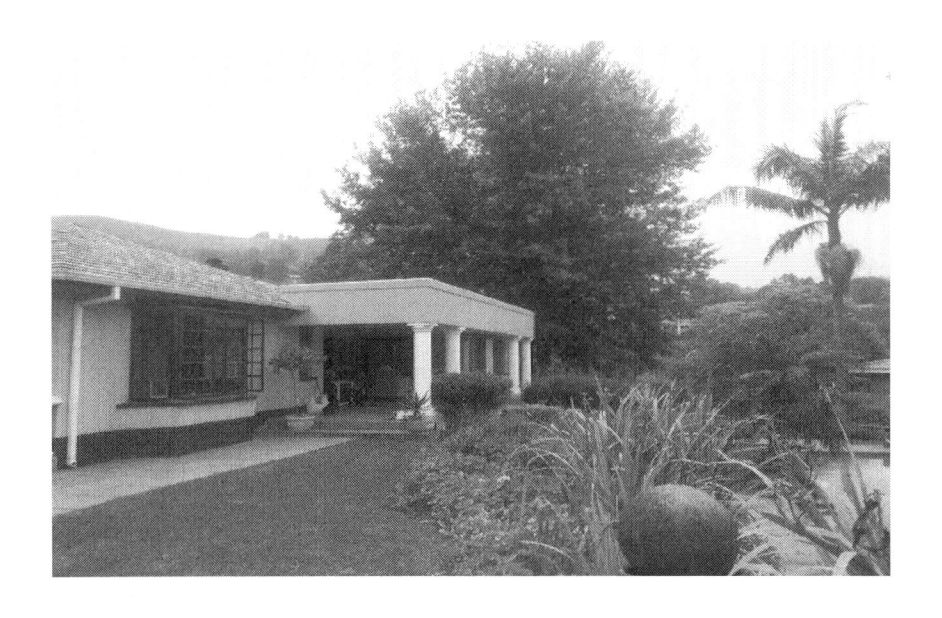

Below: This is the house we lived in when I was growing up in Pietermaritzburg. When we all moved out of home, my parents decided that it would make a great place to build a specialist facility to treat mental illness and other disorders. This will become St Catherines – building has already begun.

CHAPTER 8
LOOKING BACK

In 2000 the entire family paid a visit to Austria for a two-week skiing holiday. I was ecstatic; arriving in a foreign country, a completely different world from placid Pietermaritzburg. I loved Austria and the holiday was a complete and utter *jol* – there is no other way to describe it; from dawn until dusk, a mammoth *jol!*

I had a bright orange ski-suit (resulting in the nickname "Oros Man") and I took to the slopes like a natural. Speed was joy and although I nearly mowed down goodness knows how many people in the process, I rushed down those slopes in sheer delight.

There were green lights for go, red lights for stop, but to me all lights were green and the world was mine, all mine! The après ski was the cherry on the top after a fabulous day in the snow. My parents, armed with the latest technology video-ed the holiday and I recently replayed the entire two weeks. The video shows me being warm and witty displaying almost palpable energy, but I did not recognise the scary wild teenager that I had been.

I acted as if I owned the place and I suspect I thought I did! My commentary on the video was, even if I do say so myself, extraordinary. I had a way of expressing myself that was both witty and affectionate and I came across as loving the whole wide world.

Mom and Dad must have had some anxious moments, in fact, looking back Mom was not a regular participant in our outings and spent a lot of time reading in her room rather than joining us. The other members of my family were also a bit perplexed at my behaviour.

The Mirror has Two Faces

I was cheerfully kissing the ski instructors despite having a boyfriend back in South Africa is but one example and I flirted outrageously – I was after all completely irresistible.

I did, however, manage to behave within the social boundaries and can only think that despite being on a manic high the basic tenants and morals instilled in me were still rigorously adhered to and I didn't go dashing off in the dark with my handsome ski-instructors, but I certainly gave them the impression that I might!

In retrospect, I suspect my family were very glad that my daylight hours were spent entirely out on the slopes and just kept their fingers crossed that I wouldn't have an accident. Après ski was a little different as we were all together and I swanned around convinced I was the most alluring girl in the world.

They must have found me embarrassing. My poor brother when I blithely attempted karaoke! I still recall him tugging at my sleeve and trying to get me off the stage as I screeched incoherently into the mike. At the time it was a case of '"Everyone stands aside for Cally!' but poor Derrin was beyond embarrassed at my behaviour, but I couldn't have cared less!

Looking at the video I experienced both shock and awe. I don't really recognise the Oros Man, but strange feelings welled up in me as the video progressed. There was the jolly Cally, the one who spread love and laughter, a positive and seemingly endless supply of energy and joy, but today I cannot recognise how I felt then. There was the reckless girl on the bum board, all kitted out against the cold, ready to hurtle down the slopes, smiling, talking and joking.

Absolutely no alcohol was involved, but you would be forgiven for thinking I was teetering around with a bottle of schnapps permanently on hand! Who on earth was this girl?

Returning home however brought with it the corresponding low so characteristic of the disease.

In a few short days the Austrian ski slopes, the wild and wonderful nightlife had been replaced by terror and it was as if those two weeks had never happened.

I was back in St. Anne's forcing jelly down my throat and finding life pointless again. My mind was like a heap of rubble populated by a vast army of constantly scrabbling and squabbling rats. I had long conversations out aloud with myself and even questioned if I was insane, but couldn't decide if that was a bad thing or not.

Insane, such a catch-all word and so often incorrectly ascribed to the bipolar. Sedated I distantly heard the quiet hum of traffic and the odd toot of a horn, a world far from my own and although immobilised in a hospital bed all I wanted to do was go home and end my life as soon as possible.

Although looking at that video produced a surprising number of painful thoughts and memories, I'm truly grateful to have been able to watch it again. If other sufferers find themselves with the same opportunity, I urge them to do the same. It will not be easy, but it is an important aid to the healing process.

It brought home how far I have travelled along the rocky road to normality. Yes, it did make me sad and yes it brought back thoughts and feelings I had thought long buried and a lot of them were not very pleasant, but its therapeutic aspect cannot be denied.

How easily we forget feelings and emotions, how easy it is to view the past from the joy of the present and how easy to re-colour the bad bits into a more appealing hue. The darkness of those feelings and memories throws a spotlight on the present highlighting the achievement.

Do it if you can, you may wipe away a few tears, but you will not be disappointed and will find deeper confidence in the present. Today I can honestly say I am healed and pray to God that this healing will continue for the rest of my life.

The stark reality being that once bipolar, always bipolar, but with the resilience of myself, my family and the guidance of a loving God, I pray the rest of my days will be spent being "normal".

Defining normal, as mentioned before, is impossible, but *not* being normal is very easy to identify and God willing I will never have to back there ever again.

CHAPTER NINE

HOPE

It's been a long journey, although some of it remains a blur. Being forced to visit the darkest places in one's soul is an intensely unpleasant experience and most of us seldom dare go there consciously.

However, in those dark depths I believe is the essence of who you are and looking beneath the surface gives you an amazing opportunity and the strength to really look at yourself. No one likes a visit to the dentist with a painful aching jaw, but once the tooth is filled and the pain goes away you can't imagine why you didn't speedily and joyfully head off to the dental clinic at the first twinge in your tooth. Visiting your soul can be like that, take the courage and pay it a visit.

Throughout all these jumbled years of pain, rejection and suffering I discovered that joy and peace, which is something we all desire and aspire to, really only start when you seek to understand and confront your own inner being, your soul.

The resulting realisation that happiness and peace have nothing to do with being popular, or famous, or hugely materialistically successful, it all comes down in the end to truly knowing who you really are. Who you really are is beautiful, we are all beautiful, we just sometimes forget and let the world whisk us away into the realm of materialistic survival, leaving the beauty behind.

The whole process is humbling, no one is greater than another in the broader sense of the word. So-called 'failures' produce volumes of wisdom.

Despite the fact that your mind may be kept on an even keel by ongoing medication and care, your soul is the important one, enabling you to walk in forgiveness, joy and love.

Oh, and don't forget to cry when you need to! Don't be afraid of those tears because when you cry you are most alive that is when God's spirit is moving within you, touching you with His healing.

I know that 'normality' is a rare word for a bipolar sufferer to use, yet that is what I am feeling now. I have learnt that there is always hope amidst the chaos and confusion and even in despair one is reminded to just live another day as tomorrow might be the turning point – and one day tomorrow will come.

This I have lived, so this I know. My hope for you the reader is that you live another day where madness has no power over you, you have the power to rise above its seductive clutches and live, truly live. To be able to look into the mirror and know that happy person smiling back at you.

CHAPTER TEN
FAMILY SUPPORT

Disease of any kind is never isolated, the sufferer unwittingly sends out circles of discord to those around. When I was finally diagnosed, there was acceptance, coupled with relief, but the impact of the disease continued to influence the family for the next sixteen years. It would only be fair to offer them a chance to look at their support and let them reflect on my journey and how it affected them.

DAD
My Dad has a positive outlook on life and firmly believes good can be found in any situation – nothing stays the same forever – and he instantly accepted the challenges of my diagnosis. Dad is a realist and the only question he ever asks is "What can I do to make things better". The quote, attributed to Reinhold Niebuhr, could have been written for my father. *"God grant me the serenity to accept the things I cannot change, the courage to change the things I can and the wisdom to know the difference"*.

Dad had an unwavering belief that I would get better and lead a normal life. When he looks back on those chaotic years there are two incidents that remain firmly imprinted on his mind. The first was in the early years, long before diagnosis, when I decided to take a shower in my parent's bathroom. I turned on the water and was horrified at what I saw - blood was spraying from the shower rose, there was no water, only blood. I screamed the house down. It was the first of many manic and delusional episodes my Dad had to experience, although at the time he didn't know that it was the start of an 18 year battle for his daughter's sanity.

My Dad wonders if I remember that day in Tara in the common room of my ward when I decided to recite my own poems to anyone who was within earshot – he has never asked me about this – but it produced a wry smile, I was so entertaining!

For my father, it was never a matter of having 'to come to terms' with my condition. It was an instant acceptance of the situation knowing that, other than giving unconditional love and support, there was nothing much else he could do. My Mom possesses the most amazing compassion and love so I was guaranteed the best of care; there is no substitute for love and support.

My father also believed that he had to have faith that the professionals, the psychiatrists and the psychologists, who despite not having all the answers, had my best interests at heart. He often wondered how these professionals cope in one of the most demanding and stressful vocations imaginable.

Turning a negative into a positive, as is his nature, Dad says that learnt a lot from me during those years – tolerance and patience.

"Cally endured so much, forfeited so many things during her adolescent years, things we all take for granted, yet she is the most loving and faithful human being one could ever wish to know; a wonderful sense of humour, an infectious smile. Another endearing trait is Cally is able to laugh at herself and Suzie and I are truly blessed and proud to have such a beautiful daughter. It was, however, one helluva journey! An arduous and heart-breaking journey, but I can now say that we have our daughter back! Cally is back and we look forward to the next chapter of her life."

MOM
My Mom was initially completely devastated by my diagnosis – which had taken three long years – she had never even heard of bipolar disorder at the time!

But hot on the heels of devastation came hope; with a firm diagnosis treatment could begin.
However, I am not an only child, I have a twin sister, a little sister (who was only 10 at the time) and a big brother and my mother had concerns that their lives would be overly disrupted by my behaviour. It was a roller coaster of emotions with each and every day presenting her with another set of challenges to be overcome.

One blessing during those years, whether I was on a high, or a low, (both situations difficult and scary for anyone to witness) I was never threatening to other people, I was never angry at them. My mother's advice to people who find themselves in the same situation is simple – LOVE. Endless patience, endless love, hugs and touches and external counselling.

Mom also found a silver lining,
"Cally never gave up, she was determined to get better and live a normal life. I am privileged to be her mother; she is a very special courageous young woman. Her laughter and sense of humour are gifts from heaven and to see her now, stable, working as a paralegal, and living a normal independent life is a true gift from God. She's very untidy in her room though, but I don't think that matters one whit!"

"She is gentle, strong and loyal; her belief in God surpasses anything and her continual determination to get better and live a normal life was astounding. She was determined to get her matric, determined to pass her first year at varsity, determined to attain her massage diploma and very determined to lose weight (nearly 50ks!).

This girl is so very special – a courageous young woman and we are privileged to be her parents and family and part of her journey. I love her to end of time and onwards."

The Mirror has Two Faces

LILLA (Twin)

My twin sister, Elizabeth known as Lilla, was also relieved when I received my diagnosis, she had lost her best friend when I became sick – I had simply disappeared almost overnight and she wanted me back. For 13 years we had shared everything, and assumed this would continue, but my illness prevented that. We didn't matriculate together, we didn't go to varsity together and we didn't share all those wonderful 'firsts' people experience growing up.

Lilla took on the role of being the 'healthy, normal and successful twin' as a form of compensation, an additional pressure which also took its toll manifesting many years later when Lilla was an adult, into two bouts of clinical depression.

We were young, in our formative years and Lilla was confused by my behaviour. I once told her she was John the Baptist and I was Jesus and I really believed it. It must have been particularly bizarre for her when I suddenly decided I was no longer Cally but Kyle and donned my father's clothes.

"Cally is without a doubt the strongest person I know to have endured the torment of 18 years of her life in "hell," and to have come out victorious! Cally has a beautiful, loving, kind and gentle nature and would literally not harm a fly. Even though she has been through so much she is not bitter and has never fallen into the victim trap after losing so much of her youth. I am extremely proud of my twin sister who has had immense faith throughout and who led me to my faith after 16 years of faithfully praying for me. I have learnt to have patience and hope from Cally and to always believe in a sunnier tomorrow! I am so grateful for her healing these past 4 years and can't wait to see what Cally conquers next – watch this space! I have my best friend back! Thank you Lord."

BRIDGET

Bridget, my youngest sister was only 10 at the time my diagnosis was confirmed and spent more time with me at home than the others who had by then left for varsity. Bridget was sometimes embarrassed by me, especially if I 'misbehaved' in public or at school and became slightly resentful of the attention I was receiving. However, in retrospect, Bridget says that this also had a silver lining, making her more independent, although she relied on her friends a lot to escape what was going on at home.

Bridget was too young to understand all the ins and outs of bipolar disorder, but as she grew into adulthood she realised how daunting a task our parents had faced and how we had all weathered the storm against huge odds and emerged as a family still intact and deeply committed to each other.

One of Bridget's enduring memories, when my episodes had just started, was in the Kruger Park. I was acting very strangely and when we stopped at a view site I simply wandered off. Bridget called out and started to look for me and found me poised upon a rock. I seriously informed her that I had been summoned by demons and they had told me to jump! Poor Bridget panicked and started yelling at me and pulling me back from the edge. I thought it was a huge joke and fell about laughing! Bridget remembers the incident to this day.

"I think because her disease has been a part of my family's life for so long it gets easier to accept and cope with. The fact that she has now found a treatment that works and she has been well for a long time now is a major breakthrough for her and our family too. With age and a bit more wisdom I have more compassion and understanding for my sister."

DERRIN

My brother Derrin found my diagnosis very hard to accept. In those days there were more questions than answers and he simply couldn't understand how this could come about, or accept what was happening to his sister. I'd been such a tomboy, played cricket or tennis with him until it was too dark to see, I'd been so jolly, so normal, so much fun. Derrin simply hoped that my disease was a phase and it would quickly pass.

However, there is no quick fix and Derrin completely rejected the idea that his sister had a mental illness; he couldn't understand it and found it very difficult to witness me going through tough times. He desperately tried to help and reach out to me, but I pushed him away making him feel completely inadequate. Life was so up and down, he never knew when the next high or low would hit and just when he thought he had his sister back another episode would rock the boat.

When Derrin moved to Cape Town and I also decided it was a great idea to make a fresh start and move there myself. I stayed in a family friend's home in Claremont. One afternoonI decided to out in my yellow car and failed to return home. Derrin drove round and round the neighbourhood, but there not a sight nor sound of me and the light was fading fast and he was beginning to become seriously anxious.

I was lost AND I had run out of petrol, but luckily I walked to the nearest house and made a frantic call to my brother. Somehow I'd taken wrong turns from Claremont and had ended up on the winding road to Hout Bay! Thankfully the owners of the house gave him directions and he picked me up.

Derrin particularly remembers my suicide attempts when I overdosed on pills and landed up in hospitals having my stomach pumped. There was one occasion where no one could wake me and no one knew if I would make it.

These incidents were incredibly traumatic for the entire family as you can imagine and remain as vivid memories.

My brother remembers paying me a visit at Tara. The whole family would drive up from Pietermaritzburg as often as they could. Poor Derrin was horrified at my room, it was like a prison cell with only a mattress on the floor and he couldn't believe it was his sister living like that. However, at the time I was on a manic high and couldn't have cared less. Derrin on the other hand, who had never been exposed to seriously mentally ill people, was stunned by the experience.

Derrin slowly came to realise that when I was manic, or severely depressed, it was not the real me, he also understood that medication also played a part in affecting my personality, but he found it very difficult to see his once-vibrant sister so lethargic and only wanting to sleep her days away. I was not the sister he knew and loved.

"The real Cally, however, is the most amazing caring person with so much to offer. Cally will always find the good in anyone and is extremely mindful of others. One thing for sure is she loves our family and would do anything for us."

Like all my family, Derrin too found a lesson in my illness; he says that he learnt that if you put your mind to something it can be achieved, no matter how difficult the circumstances.

"Cally has successfully come to terms with her bipolar illness and found a way to live her life to the fullest. I am immensely proud of my sister for the strength to keep going day by day and her loving and caring nature despite all she has gone through in life. There will be moments, days, weeks and months when you feel like you can't go on, but NO matter what don't lose hope."

The enduring advice to other sufferers from all my family members who have witnessed my problem from the start to the present day highlights unconditional support and love.

Read as much as possible about the condition and above all do not be ashamed, mental illness is like a physical illness and it is far more common than one realises. Family members must also support one another, its importance must never be underestimated; lean on each other and know that things will get better. Human beings are stronger than we know and the human spirit can overcome almost anything.

"....never give up on Faith in God even when times are hard and don't make sense."

There are also the subtle indicators which people can adopt making a huge emotional difference to both the sufferer and their family. Small things like a family member HAS bipolar, not IS bipolar. It is a small interesting psychological shift, but it makes a huge difference – if you have something it can be removed, but if you are something, that is a different matter.

The fact that today I have had a few jobs and am able to function as a normal adult. I worked as a paralegal with my twin sister for a while. I did administrative tasks and have also done a stint as an au pair. I lead a fully functional and independent life is due entirely to the support of my family and who worked closely with the professionals.

My parent's deep faith was (and remains) the rock to which they are anchored enabling them to weather the storms I unwittingly unleashed upon them and my siblings.

CHAPTER ELEVEN
MEDICAL MEMOIRS

DR MARIA DOBREVA'S ENCOUNTERS WITH CALLY BASSAGE

I have known Cally since her teens, which means it's nearly 20 years. I initially attended to her at Town Hill outpatients Clinic and later on in my private practice.

She was complicated and almost "Treatment Resistant" Bipolar case. I have spent many hours with Cally; regular follow-ups and assessments. Challenging and difficult times. Her moods: highs, lows or mixed. As I settled her from a manic episode, she would fall into severe depression, notoriously difficult to treat in bipolar patients. No matter how dysfunctional, distressed or even psychotic, Cally would always try and make sense of her 'reality.' It is hard to rationalise pathology in patients also tend to become psychotic, as it doesn't necessarily make sense to them and it can perhaps create unwarranted distress.

She was always eager to tease out where the symptoms came from and make sense of her feelings, moods and perceptions. I tried to explain that there wasn't necessarily a link to the unconscious mind or a case of "faulty" thinking, it is a biological illness. I clarified by trying to make her understand that mental illness is not much different from any other medical condition, except that it affects the brain function.

As if it wasn't bad enough, to suffer from Bipolar, she also had distressing OCD, paralysed by obsessive, intrusive images and thoughts of harming her loved ones.

This left her feeling distressed, ashamed and "confused." She was horrified that she would act on these thoughts, yet she never did.

So it carried on for years; in and out of hospitals, trials of various mood stabilisers, anti-depressants and antipsychotics, hours in psychotherapy. Cally's life was a string of ups and downs and chaos; many golden job opportunities, many changes and many failures.

However, unlike many others in her predicament, Cally never gave up. She went on fighting and holding on to the hope that things will get better one day. It was that unbreakable spirit of staying positive and hopeful that helped her pull through, and after many years of trials and errors, we finally got the medication cocktail right some three years ago.

What an amazing success story. I look at Cally now and I can hardly believe that she has endured nearly 20 years of absolute "Hell." She is fully functional and enjoys a happy and healthy relationship with her family and friends.

It has been and remains an absolute privilege to have walked this walk with Cal and help her to where she is now.

I am so proud of you Cally.

CHAPTER TWELVE

LIVING IN THE NOW

Things began to change for me in 2013. I had suffered from bipolar depression for so many years that at times it felt as if this was going to be my life. One minute I was living a relatively normal existence but always the fear of the darkness was hiding inside. I could not trust that a month or weeks into the future I would still be fine.

My life was almost suspended. I could not make concrete plans for fear that I would go plunging into the abyss. I had dreams of how I would like to live but always these dreams and goals were tinged with – "What if I am not better? What if I have another episode?"

I think one of the hardest things in the recovery process is to trust yourself and to get to know your moods, thoughts and feelings. After years of living with bipolar, I knew when I started to feel unsettled. I could tell the difference between a normal bad day and the possible onset of a bad depressive episode. I was learning to tune into my body and its responses.

At times in the past, I felt that I had to pretend that everything was alright. I would sense an emotional wobble and then I would think that I could will the illness away. I did not want my parents to worry about me all the time. But suppressing these symptoms would invariably make them worse.

I learnt that it was vital for me to be honest about my feelings and to immediately consult a doctor when I felt I was losing equilibrium.

My family were also good at judging my moods and behaviour and sometimes they were more attuned than I was, asking how I felt and if I was okay.

It is a double-edged sword – because you appreciate that they care about you but you also resent them for their constant concern and worry.

For me the turning point was in 2013 when I was introduced to a new medication... I had been seeing Dr Salduker, a psychiatrist in Durban for a year or two and I had been able to live my life reasonably well with only the odd bipolar episode.

He suggested that I try **_Risperdal*_**. It was a new drug that was used for bipolar but also it was helpful in treating patients who suffered from hallucinations. I had been diagnosed as possibly having border-line schizophrenia, as I sometimes had vivid hallucinations when I was in a full-blown manic episode.

Dr Dobreva suggested that I try a drug called **_Xeplion*_** that was new on the market and it was expensive. It has to be administered via a monthly injection and the effects monitored closely to see if it was the correct dosage.

I was on a number of medications to stabilise my condition was always at some point it seemed their effectiveness wore off. In difficult bipolar cases, the body becomes medication resistant and the effectiveness of the drugs wear off. But the Xeplion injections were to change my life.

For the first time, I was able to feel confident and stable. I was even able to see further than next week and I felt excited to make plans to get a job and to re-build my life. I no longer lived with the constant fear of a bipolar episode interrupting my life.

I had lived half of my adult life with bipolar and for 15 years it had seemed as though my life was a runaway train. Suddenly I was able to think clearly and to feel "normal".

In the past three years, I have made great strides in my recovery. For some people getting a job and having a boyfriend are normal everyday events. But for me bipolar had always made me scared of committing to something that I might ruin.

Trying a variety of medications had also wreaked havoc with my body. I had put on a huge amount of weight (a common side effect) and my poor health had been an excuse for me to avoid regular exercise and to binge on junk food.

I decided that I needed to take control of my body and my weight and I embarked on a banting diet. I focused on eating protein and vegetables and cutting back on carbohydrates. I also investigated whether this diet would have any negative side effects, all the doctors said that losing weight would have an all-round positive effect.

It was hard work but I stuck to the diet and over the course of 18 months, I lost 48 kilograms. I t was proof that if I set my mind to something I could achieve it.

In 2016 I met a man who would become an important part of my life. Greg and I were part of the same church community and when he learned of my bipolar he never judged me. We became friends and we shared a love of soccer and were both family-oriented.

Soon after Christmas 2016, we started dating. I was 33-years-old and suddenly I was sharing my life with someone who saw me as Cally – a normal woman. He was supportive and would go with me to the chemist to get my ***Xeplion*** injections.

He read up a lot on bipolar. It didn't put him off me and I finally found someone who saw me for more than a person suffering from bipolar.

We really enjoy each other's company and he has become an important part of my life. We have common values and we are both committed Christians.

Today I do a few part-time jobs and every day I am learning skills and growing in confidence. Skills that people take for granted like computer skills were not part of my life – I had a lot of catching up to do.

One of the hardest issues for me was to learn to relax around people in social situations. A bipolar sufferer is often only in the company of their family or medical professionals and the small talk that seems to come naturally to others is hard for us.

I lived so much according to regimens that were designed to make me live "normally" that it was hard for me to be spontaneous and enjoy fun things.

Working at the law firm made me realise how to relax and to socialise and to develop an identity that wasn't "Cally – the bipolar". I learnt how to laugh at small things and to have opinions and most of all I learnt not to be so hard on myself if I made mistakes.

It has been a process of re-discovering who I am and also looking forward to developing into a new person who no longer feels afraid. It is the fear that holds us back in life and no longer living in fear of regular relapses into bipolar means I can explore a whole new world.

I am now able to plan into the future and have some certainty that things will work out. Nothing in life is ever absolutely certain ... but taking small steps forward every day means I am moving in the right direction.

CHAPTER THIRTEEN

ADVICE & RESOURCES

HOW DO YOU KNOW IF YOU ARE BIPOLAR?

Highs are periods of mania, while lows are periods of depression. The mood swings may even become mixed so you might feel elated and depressed at the same time. Bipolar disorder can be hard to diagnose but there are warning signs or symptoms that you can look for.

WHAT IS THE DIFFERENCE BETWEEN BIPOLAR AND DEPRESSION?

The main difference between bipolar disorder and depression are the main symptoms characterised by excessive excitement or irritability, extreme elation and delusions of grandeur that are associated with the bipolar condition.

HOW DO I KNOW IF MY BIPOLAR MEDS ARE WORKING?

Whenever you take psychiatric medication, research it and know what it is supposed to do. This means understanding the target symptoms it is intended to affect. How long is it suppose to take to feel the full effect? Will you have to try several different medications or a combination if you're not feeling better?

. Know about your medication read the instructions, side effects and interactions

. Be honest about your medication compliance

. It is possible to tell if your symptoms are better

. Evaluate the recovery process itself

CAN A GENERAL PRACTITIONER TREAT BIPOLAR?

If you're already taking medication for bipolar disorder and you develop depression your GP will check you're taking the correct dose. Episodes of depression are treated slightly differently in bipolar disorder as the use of antidepressants alone may lead to a hypomanic relapse.

WHAT DO I DO IF I AM FEELING AN EPISODE COMING?

No matter how down or out of control you feel it's important to remember that you are not powerless when it comes to bipolar disorder. Beyond the treatment you get from your doctor or therapist there are many things you can do to reduce your symptoms and stay on track, including educating yourself about bipolar disorder. Don't panic!

WHERE CAN I GET SUPPORT FOR MY BIPOLAR?

Doctors almost always prescribe medication for people with bipolar disorder. Just talking with a therapist isn't enough to control bipolar disorder, especially during episodes of mania or depression. There is a huge need for bipolar support groups. A bipolar sufferer must surround herself/himself with loved ones, family and friends. Do not isolate yourself!

MY FAMILY DON'T UNDERSTAND ... HOW CAN I EXPLAIN MY CONDITION?

STEP 1: Remain calm and non-defensive. As frustrating as it was that my loved ones didn't understand my illness I had to keep in mind that at first I didn't understand either. You're in the role of teacher and the person you're talking to is a student.

STEP 2: Give them the official definition and credit the source.

STEP 3: Tell them the story of how you came to be diagnosed with bipolar disorder.

CAN BIPOLAR BE CURED?

Research has shown there is no known cure for bipolar disorder but symptoms can be managed with a combination of psychiatric medication and psychotherapy.

WHAT ACTIVITIES HELPED YOU DURING YOUR ILLNESS?

. Writing- expressing my thoughts and feelings through writing poetry and writing in my journal

. Exercising- walking/running, cycling, breathing in the fresh air!

. Sun therapy- having enough vitamin D

. Eating a low - carb diet- low in sugar and high in fats have been proven very beneficial for mental health patients. (The Banting Diet)

.Sometimes reading but mostly during a depressed state.

IS THERE A SUPPORT GROUP FOR PEOPLE WITH BIPOLAR?

SADAG - South African Depression and Anxiety Group

www.sadag.org.za

HOW CAN FAMILIES HELP A MEMBER WHO HAS BIPOLAR?

If someone you love has a mood disorder you may be feeling helpless, overwhelmed, confused and hopeless or you may feel hurt angry, frustrated and resentful. Be patient, kind and tolerant towards your bipolar family member. Give love and support. Be alert for any dangerous, life-threatening tendencies/symptoms-suicide etc.

CAN I BE DISCRIMINATED AGAINST AT WORK IF I TELL MY EMPLOYERS I HAVE BIPOLAR?

A bipolar disorder diagnosis can have a big effect on your job or career. If you need to take time off because of your bipolar disorder see if your employer has disability insurance or look into Social Security Disability insurance. You don't have to talk to your boss or co-workers about your bipolar disorder. But if your condition has been affecting your performance at work, being open may be a good idea. Your boss and co-workers may have noticed the changes in your behaviour. If you explain what's going on they may be more sympathetic and helpful than you expect.

WHAT TRIGGERS BIPOLAR?

Hormonal problems: Hormonal imbalances might trigger or cause bipolar disorder.

Environmental factors: Abuse, mental stress, a "significant loss" or some other traumatic event may contribute to triggering bipolar disorder.

GLOSSARY

This is a list of the medical terms/ medicines that are referred to in this book. Please consult a medical professional before asking for any of these medicines. They have different uses for different situations. Finding the correct balance is vital in coping with bipolar disorder and what works for one person may not work for another.

Ativan: A tranquilizer and sedative
Urbanol: mild anxiolytics/tranquilizer
Epilium: mood stabilizer
Lithium: mood stabilizer
Serdep: an antidepressant (SSRI)
Topomax: mood stabalizer
Clozapine: anti-psychotic
Risperdal: injection-anti psychotic medication
Xeplion: injection-antipsychotic medication
Eltroxin: a thyroid supplement

POETRY

I often used to write poetry to try and work out my thoughts and feelings. It was a useful tool to put onto paper what was happening in my head. Later I began to write a comprehensive diary/book. I would recommend it as one of the tools to help.

I have included here some of the poems I think best describe what I was going through.

My Family

*They know you
through and through.*

*Through the good times and the bad.
They are there.*

*Eyes peering at you,
from in front of you,
besides you,
and even behind.*

*They will catch you
when you fall.
and support you,
until you are well again.*

Until it happens once again.

*My family,
my support.*
_ Cally Bassage

The Mirror has Two Faces

"Living to the Ultimate"

Living to the ultimate,
Dancing on water,
Never looking back
I hear her, this small-child like voice- "Come
Nearer, nearer still, I love you.
I need you, don't leave me."

Living to the ultimate,
Racing thoughts,
Beautiful dreams and
Aspirations
People everywhere,
Laughing,
Dancing,
Singing the old tunes,
"I love you, I need you don't leave me today"

"The mirror has two faces,"
Night vs day
Black vs white
Smiles vs frown
Highs vs lows

"Bipolar," is the word the professionals have labelled me,
the stigmatic sting of the word piercing into my heart.
It follows me so closely and in an impulse
strangles, suffocating the life of me.

And then the creativity,
The brightness of a rainbow of colours.
So pure, so innocent, so raw.
Leading me,
Guiding me to
The ultimate.

Darkness finds me

Darkness all around me,
Looming in the ally ways
Creeping up behind me
Infront of me
and alongside me,
Where to run to,
Where to hide,
Take me away from this inflicting hell,
it rots and gnaws at my bones
at the marrow of my bones,
A cry for help
No one, nobody can hear me
but only you
The darkness all around.

- Cally Bassage

Medical miracles

They are called the Professionals.

The one's we like to call doctors, psychiatrists, psychologists and nurses,

Although they are not God,

They hold my existence in their grasp.

One decision- it could fail

One decision- it could prosper.

A hit and miss

A cat and mouse game,

My Doctor- compassionate and kind,

Being patient after all those years.

A hope, a light in the darkness,

A light, a hope for greater things,

My miracle,

My xeplion injection!

-Cally Bassage

ABOUT THE AUTHOR

Cally Bassage became ill in her early teens and went through years of mental anguish as she went from doctors to psychiatrists trying to figure out what was wrong with her. In her late teens she was diagnosed with bipolar disorder and has been trying to manage her life with this unpredictable and challenging condition.
In this book she explains how bipolar disorder affects her life and how she has managed to get through some very scary times. Today she has her condition under control but her journey has taught her that family support and education is so crucial to helping people understand what she is experiencing.
Today she lives between Ballito and Pietermaritzburg in South Africa and has a few part time jobs. She hopes that by telling her story she will be able to give hope to others who may be experiencing the same situation and also she hopes to offer talks to any group, church or community that are interested in hearing about her experience with bipolar disorder.

Website: www.callybassage.co.za
Email: callybookmail@gmail.com

Made in the USA
Middletown, DE
28 October 2020